Liver Cirrhosis Treatment and Diet

For Newly Diagnosed

Reverse Fatty Liver Disease, Heal the Immune System, and Eliminate Toxins with These Liver Healing Diet Meal Recipes.

TABLE OF CONTENT

INTRODUCTION

A cirrhosis diet is intended to support those with the disease who may experience malnourishment as a result of altered digestion and metabolism brought on by increased liver impairment.

What you eat and drink daily is particularly crucial if you have cirrhosis. Protein, sodium, and sugar are included in many foods that are best avoided if you have cirrhosis because they make your liver work harder, which may eventually wear it down.

This book describes how to work with your healthcare team, including a certified dietitian, to create a cirrhosis diet plan. By doing this, you can make sure that you're getting enough nutrition and steer clear of decisions that could make your health worse or have other negative effects.

Understanding Liver Cirrhosis

Cirrhosis of the liver is a chronic and irreversible disease of the liver that is defined by the replacement of good liver tissue by scar tissue resulting from the condition. The normal structure of the liver is disrupted as a result of this scarring, which in turn hinders the liver's ability to operate normally. The liver is a multifunctional organ that plays a significant part in a variety of physiological processes. These functions include metabolism, detoxification, and the creation of proteins that are utilized in the process of blood coagulation. Cirrhosis is a condition that prevents these vital functions from functioning properly, which can result in a variety of issues.

Definition and Causes

Liver cirrhosis usually appears gradually, frequently as a result of ongoing liver disease. Understanding the several causes of cirrhosis is essential for both effective care and prevention.

Alcohol-Associated Hepatic Cirrhosis: A major contributing factor to cirrhosis is alcohol abuse. Over time, chronic alcohol misuse causes the liver tissue to become inflamed and scarred, which eventually leads to cirrhosis. To avoid alcohol-related liver damage, people must be informed of acceptable alcohol consumption guidelines.

Chronic Viral Hepatitis: Viral infections such as hepatitis B and C can cause persistent liver inflammation, which can hasten the onset of cirrhosis. It is essential to comprehend the methods of transmission, available vaccinations, and early detection of viral hepatitis to prevent and treat cirrhosis in these situations.

Alcohol use has no connection to the accumulation of fat in the liver which is the hallmark of non-alcoholic fatty liver disease (NAFLD). Obesity, insulin resistance, and metabolic syndrome are frequently linked to NAFLD. Preventing and treating NAFLD-related cirrhosis primarily involves controlling weight and leading a healthy lifestyle.

Stages of Liver Cirrhosis

There are various phases of liver cirrhosis, and each one indicates the degree of liver damage. Comprehending these phases is essential for medical practitioners to identify suitable therapeutic approaches and for patients to grasp the possible influence on their well-being.

Compensated cirrhosis: In the early stages, there may not be many symptoms and the liver may still be able to carry out its vital tasks. Nonetheless, there is a great deal of scarring, and further development must be stopped by interventions.

Decompensated Cirrhosis: As the disease progresses, the liver's capacity to function deteriorates, which can result in consequences such as variceal hemorrhage, hepatic encephalopathy, ascites, or an accumulation of fluid in the abdomen. Decompensated cirrhosis may need a liver transplant and calls for more stringent medical care.

End-Stage Cirrhosis: The liver has suffered significant damage and is significantly compromised in its ability to operate. The main course of treatment for end-stage cirrhosis is liver transplantation.

Importance of Diet in Treatment

Diet has a complex function in the therapy of liver cirrhosis; it is important for symptom management, disease progression slowing, and liver health maintenance. A well-planned diet can have a positive impact on the lives of people with cirrhosis.

Handling Malnutrition: People with liver cirrhosis often worry about malnutrition because of things like decreased appetite, weakened nutrient absorption, and higher energy use. Malnutrition must be prevented and treated with a well-balanced diet full of important nutrients to assist the body's healing processes.

Protein Intake and Ammonia Levels: When the liver is injured, the metabolic byproduct of protein metabolism, ammonia, builds up in the blood. Keeping protein intake under control is crucial for treating symptoms such as hepatic encephalopathy, particularly when it comes to meals high in ammonia.

Limiting Sodium: Ascites, or the buildup of fluid in the abdomen, is a frequent side effect of cirrhosis. Limiting salt consumption aids in the control of fluid retention and the reduction of ascite symptoms.

Macronutrient Balancing: For people with cirrhosis, maintaining a balance between proteins, carbs, and fats is essential. This equilibrium upholds energy needs, assists in preserving a healthy weight, and enhances general well-being.

Micronutrients and Antioxidants: A sufficient diet rich in vitamins and minerals, including selenium, and vitamins C, and E, helps protect liver cells from oxidative stress. Foods high in antioxidants help to maintain liver health and reduce inflammation.

CHAPTER 1: BASICS OF LIVER HEALTH

The liver is a fascinating organ that plays a crucial part in ensuring that the body's state of health and well-being is maintained throughout its entirety. The complex nature of its structure and the fact that it can perform multiple functions make it an essential component in a variety of physiological processes. The architecture and function of the liver, as well as its involvement in digestion and its vital role in detoxification processes, are discussed in this section. Additionally, an overview of common liver disorders, such as hepatitis, fatty liver disease, and cirrhosis, is provided.

Anatomy and Function of the Liver

- **The Liver's Role in Digestion**

The liver is situated immediately below the diaphragm in the upper right section of the abdominal cavity. It has two main lobes and is the largest internal organ. It has a special blood supply because it gets blood from the portal vein, which gets blood rich in nutrients from the digestive organs, and the hepatic artery, which gets blood that is oxygenated.

The processing and distribution of nutrients throughout the body are critically dependent on the liver's role in digestion. The liver metabolizes and stores nutrients as blood from the digestive organs passes through the portal vein. It is essential for the metabolism of fat, protein, and carbohydrates.

Carbohydrate Metabolism: By storing extra glucose as glycogen and releasing it when the body needs energy, the liver aids in controlling blood glucose levels. This guarantees that the brain and other organs will always have access to glucose.

Protein Metabolism: The liver produces the clotting components required for healthy blood coagulation as well as proteins like albumin, which aids in maintaining blood pressure and volume.

Fat Metabolism: Bile, a chemical essential to fat digestion and absorption, is produced by the liver. When necessary, bile is expelled from the gallbladder and placed into the small intestine. The liver also contributes to the creation of lipoproteins, which are responsible for carrying fats through the bloodstream.

- **Detoxification Processes**

Because it is so important in the removal of waste materials and toxins from the body, the liver is frequently referred to as the detoxification center. Hazardous substances are changed during this process into compounds that are soluble in water and can be eliminated through bile or urine.

Phase I Detoxification: Toxins are broken down by the liver's enzymes, which also increase their solubility in water and set them up for subsequent processing.

Phase II Detoxification: Additional changes are made to water-soluble chemicals, such as conjugation with molecules like glutathione, which facilitates their excretion.

Maintaining a healthy internal environment and shielding the body from the damaging effects of drugs, pollutants, and metabolic byproducts are made possible by the liver's detoxification processes.

Common Liver Conditions

- **Hepatitis**

Hepatitis is an inflammatory disease of the liver that is typically brought on by viral infections, although it can also be brought on by autoimmune reactions, drug exposure, or environmental pollutants. Hepatitis A, B, and C are the most common viral hepatitis kinds, while there are other varieties as well.

Hepatitis A: Usually acute and not associated with chronic liver disease, hepatitis A is spread by tainted food and water. For prevention, vaccination is an option.

Hepatitis B: Can cause chronic infection and raise the risk of cirrhosis and liver cancer, it is spread via contact with contaminated blood or bodily fluids or by an infected mother giving birth to her child. Vaccination is a successful preventative strategy.

Hepatitis C: Mostly spread via blood contact, this infection frequently results in chronic infection and can advance to cirrhosis and liver cancer. Hepatitis C cannot be prevented, however, antiviral drugs can be used as a treatment.

- **Fatty Liver Disease**

The disorder known as Non-Alcoholic Fatty Liver Disease (NAFLD) is typified by the buildup of fat in the liver that is not connected to binge drinking. It includes a range of liver diseases, from non-alcoholic steatohepatitis (NASH), which causes inflammation and destruction of the liver cells, to plain fatty liver (steatosis).

Common risk factors for non-alcoholic fatty liver disease (NAFLD) include obesity, insulin resistance, type 2 diabetes, high blood pressure, and metabolic syndrome. A balanced diet and weight loss are two important lifestyle changes for controlling and avoiding NAFLD.

- **Cirrhosis Overview**

Cirrhosis represents the advanced stage of liver fibrosis, characterized by the irreversible scarring of liver tissue. Chronic liver damage, often stemming from conditions such as chronic alcohol consumption, viral hepatitis, or fatty liver disease, can lead to cirrhosis.

Progression of Cirrhosis: In the early stages, the liver attempts to repair itself, leading to the formation of scar tissue. As cirrhosis progresses, the liver's structure becomes distorted, impairing its function. Complications such as portal hypertension, ascites, hepatic encephalopathy, and an increased risk of liver cancer can arise.

Symptoms of Cirrhosis: Early stages may be asymptomatic, but as cirrhosis advances, symptoms such as fatigue, weakness, easy bruising, swelling in the legs and abdomen, and confusion may manifest.

Treatment and Management: While cirrhosis is irreversible, early intervention can slow its progression and manage complications. Treatment may involve addressing the underlying cause, lifestyle modifications, medications, and in severe cases, liver transplantation.

CHAPTER 2: CAUSES AND RISK FACTORS OF LIVER CIRRHOSIS

Cirrhosis of the liver is a dangerous disorder that worsens over time and is indicated by the formation of scar tissue in the liver that cannot be removed. Even though the liver possesses a remarkable capacity for regeneration, persistent injury and inflammation can eventually result in fibrosis and cirrhosis to develop. In the following part, we will discuss the numerous causes and risk factors that are connected with liver cirrhosis. These include alcohol-related liver cirrhosis, chronic viral hepatitis (especially Hepatitis B and C), and non-alcoholic fatty liver disease (NAFLD).

Alcohol-Related Liver Cirrhosis

- **Safe Alcohol Consumption Guidelines**

One major factor contributing to liver cirrhosis is excessive alcohol use. Alcohol is metabolized by the liver, and heavy and chronic drinking can overload the liver's processing ability, causing scarring and inflammation.

Safe Alcohol Consumption Guidelines: People must abide by these recommendations to avoid alcohol-related liver damage. Though there are differences in definitions, "safe" drinking usually refers to moderate alcohol consumption. One drink for women and two for men per day is commonly considered to be moderate drinking. Five ounces of wine, twelve ounces of beer, or 1.5 ounces of distilled spirits contain about 14 grams of pure alcohol or one standard drink.

It is imperative to comprehend and adhere to these guidelines to prevent liver cirrhosis caused by alcohol. People can evaluate and address their alcohol consumption in the context of their overall health with the assistance of regular medical check-ups and open communication with healthcare providers.

Chronic Viral Hepatitis

Viral hepatitis is a category of viral diseases that mostly damage the liver. Hepatitis B and C are the most prominent culprits in the development of chronic liver disease, including cirrhosis. Viral hepatitis is a group of diseases that are transmitted by viruses.

- **Hepatitis B**

Transmission of the viral infection known as hepatitis B occurs when an individual comes into touch with infected blood or other bodily fluids. The development of cirrhosis is a potential consequence of chronic hepatitis B infection.

Prevention and Vaccination: Getting vaccinated against hepatitis B and the eventual development of liver cirrhosis is one of the most effective strategies to avoid the disease. It is suggested that those who are at risk, such as those who work in healthcare, those who have several sexual partners, and those who live in areas with a high frequency of hepatitis B, get vaccinated.

- **Hepatitis C**

Exposure to infected blood is the primary means by which hepatitis C is transmitted. This infection is typically transmitted through the sharing of needles, risky medical practices, or the receipt of tainted blood products before the widespread deployment of screening. One of the most significant risk factors for liver cirrhosis is a chronic infection with hepatitis C.

In particular, screening for hepatitis C is essential for persons who have a history of intravenous drug use or other risk factors. Antiviral treatment is also an important component of the screening process. To treat hepatitis C and lower the likelihood of developing cirrhosis, antiviral medicines are already available. The advancement of liver disease to a more advanced stage can be prevented with early detection and treatment.

Non-Alcoholic Fatty Liver Disease (NAFLD)

Non-alcoholic fatty Liver Disease (NAFLD) is a wide term that comprises a variety of disorders that are defined by the buildup of fat in the liver. These terms are used interchangeably. The presence of non-alcoholic fatty liver disease (NAFLD) is a significant factor in the development of liver cirrhosis and is frequently linked to metabolic variables.

- **Obesity and Metabolic Syndrome**

Two of the main risk factors for the onset and course of NAFLD are obesity and metabolic syndrome. The buildup of fat in the liver is directly associated with excess body weight, particularly in the abdominal area.

Insulin Resistance: The condition in which the body's cells become less sensitive to insulin is frequently linked to obesity and metabolic syndrome. NAFLD is a result of fat being stored in the liver due to insulin resistance.

- **Importance of Weight Management**

Lifestyle Changes: Since obesity, metabolic syndrome, and non-alcoholic fatty liver disease are closely related, controlling one's weight is essential to both avoiding and treating liver cirrhosis. A balanced diet and regular exercise are two key lifestyle changes that help people reach and stay at a healthy weight.

Dietary Strategies: You can improve the health of your liver by eating a diet high in fruits, vegetables, whole foods, and lean proteins and reducing your intake of processed foods and added sugars. Mindful eating and portion control help manage weight and lower the chance of NAFLD developing further.

Physical Activity: Maintaining a healthy weight is aided by regular physical activity, which also enhances insulin sensitivity and supports overall metabolic health. It has been demonstrated that strength training and aerobic exercise help lower the incidence of liver cirrhosis linked to nonalcoholic fatty liver disease (NAFLD).

CHAPTER 3: MEDICAL TREATMENT APPROACHES

It is necessary to take a diverse approach to the treatment of liver cirrhosis because it is a disorder that is both complex and progressing. To ease symptoms, control the underlying causes of cirrhosis, and either prevent or treat consequences, medical interventions are being implemented by medical professionals. In this part, a complete description of medical treatment techniques is provided. These treatments include drugs such as antiviral medications and immunosuppressants, as well as surgical therapies such as liver transplants and shunt procedures.

Medications for Liver Cirrhosis

- **Antiviral Medications**

Antiviral drugs are essential for the treatment of liver cirrhosis, especially when a chronic viral infection like hepatitis B or C is the underlying cause of the disease.

Antiviral Therapy for Hepatitis B: Liver cirrhosis might worsen as a result of a persistent Hepatitis B infection. Antiviral drugs like tenofovir and entecavir are frequently administered to prevent viral replication, lessen inflammation, and moderate liver damage. To evaluate the efficacy of treatment, liver function, and viral load must be regularly monitored.

Antiviral Therapy for Hepatitis C: Direct-acting antiviral (DAA) drugs, which are extremely effective and well-tolerated, have revolutionized the field of Hepatitis C treatment. These medications stop the progression of liver damage and have a high cure rate because they specifically target certain stages of the Hepatitis C viral lifecycle. Individual cases determine the length of the course of treatment and the particular drugs to be used, and frequent check-ins are made to assess how well the treatment is working.

- **Immunosuppressants**

Immunosuppressive drugs may be used when cirrhosis is linked to autoimmune liver disorders. These medications work by modifying the immune system to lessen inflammation and delay the deterioration of liver damage.

Treatment for Autoimmune Hepatitis: The immune system wrongly attacking liver cells is the hallmark of autoimmune hepatitis. This immune response is frequently suppressed by immunosuppressants such as azathioprine and corticosteroids (prednisone). Effective management of the illness requires regular monitoring of liver function and dosage adjustments for medications.

Liver transplantation immunosuppression: Immunosuppressive drugs play a vital role in the post-transplant care of patients undergoing liver transplantation. These medications balance the risk of infection and other side effects with the ability to stop the immune system from rejecting the transplanted liver. The patient's medical history, reaction to treatment, and other factors are taken into consideration while selecting and dosing immunosuppressants.

Surgical Interventions

- **Liver Transplantation**

When all other therapeutic options have failed and the liver's function is seriously impaired, liver transplantation is the only surgical surgery left for end-stage liver cirrhosis. The intricate process entails removing the damaged liver and replacing it with a healthy donor liver.

Indications for Liver Transplantation: Prospects for liver transplantation undergo a meticulous selection process that takes into account several factors such as the degree of liver disease, general well-being, and the probability of a successful transplant. Hepatocellular carcinoma, liver failure, and decompensated cirrhosis are common indications (liver cancer).

Donor Options: Living or deceased donors may be used in liver transplants. Organs from deceased people whose organs are still viable for transplantation are used in deceased donor transplantation. A part of a healthy person's liver is removed during a living donor transplant procedure, and the liver then regenerates in both the donor and the recipient.

Post-Transplant Care: Meticulous post-operative care is essential for the successful outcome of liver transplantation. Immunosuppressive drugs are used to stop organ rejection, and patients are closely observed to identify and manage any possible side effects. For many people with end-stage cirrhosis, liver transplantation has proven to be a life-saving strategy despite its complications.

- **Shunt Procedures**

By opening a channel for blood to avoid the liver, shunt operations lower the portal vein's pressure, which is a typical symptom of severe cirrhosis and is known as portal hypertension.

Transjugular Intrahepatic Portosystemic Shunt (TIPS): This shunt technique involves severing the portal vein and hepatic vein to avoid the liver. This lessens problems like ascites and variceal hemorrhage and helps to relieve pressure in the portal vein.

TIPS Indications: When medicine and lifestyle modifications have failed to control problems from portal hypertension, TIPS is usually explored as a last resort. For those with cirrhosis, it can be a useful strategy for managing symptoms and enhancing quality of life.

Dangers and Things to Think About: Although TIPS can be useful, there are some risks involved. Hepatic encephalopathy, shunt stenosis or occlusion, and other problems that need constant observation and care are examples of potential consequences.

CHAPTER 4: NUTRITIONAL STRATEGIES FOR LIVER HEALTH

To effectively manage liver health, it is of the utmost importance to properly maintain sufficient nutrition, particularly for persons who have been diagnosed with liver cirrhosis. The maintenance of healthy liver function, the management of symptoms, and the prevention of problems can all be significantly aided by a nutritionally sound diet. The role of diet in liver cirrhosis is discussed in this section. Particular attention is paid to the significance of maintaining a well-balanced diet, the specific nutrient requirements for liver health are outlined, and dietary guidelines that are specifically designed to meet the requirements of individuals who have liver cirrhosis are

provided.

The Role of Diet in Liver Cirrhosis

- **Importance of a Balanced Diet**

For those with liver cirrhosis, a balanced diet is crucial to supplying the nutrients required for both optimal liver function and general health. A balanced diet helps promote liver function, control symptoms, and prevent malnutrition. The liver is essential to many metabolic activities.

Energy Requirements: Because of things like inflammation, a higher metabolic rate, and the body's attempts to heal injured tissues, people with liver cirrhosis frequently require more energy. Intake of sufficient calories is essential for maintaining energy balance and preventing malnutrition.

Protein Synthesis: The liver is in charge of this process, and keeping up a sufficient protein intake is crucial to avoiding muscle atrophy and promoting general tissue healing. However, depending on the person's health and the existence of issues such as hepatic encephalopathy, the kind and quantity of protein taken may need to be changed.

Micronutrient Support: A healthy diet is necessary to provide the vitamins and minerals that are important for liver function. Inadequate intake of specific nutrients can worsen liver impairment and negatively impact general health.

- ## **Nutrient Requirements for Liver Health**

Protein: Because it helps heal damaged tissue, maintains liver function, and prevents muscular atrophy, protein is essential for those with liver cirrhosis. However, ammonia is produced by the liver's breakdown of proteins and can be hazardous for those who have cirrhosis. Consequently, depending on the severity of liver illness and the existence of consequences such as hepatic encephalopathy, protein intake needs to be evaluated and modified.

Essentially, carbohydrates are a necessary form of energy. Eating foods high in complex carbs, like whole grains, fruits, and vegetables, promotes stable blood sugar levels and long-lasting energy. People with cirrhosis need to keep an eye on their carbohydrate intake, particularly if they have diabetes or insulin resistance.

Fats: Monounsaturated and polyunsaturated fats, which are included in avocados, olive oil, and fatty fish, are examples of healthy fats that can promote liver health. On the other hand, excessive consumption of trans and saturated fats should be avoided as it may worsen non-alcoholic fatty liver disease (NAFLD), a condition that frequently precedes cirrhosis.

Minerals and vitamins: A healthy liver depends on consuming enough of these nutrients. Vitamins C and E, for instance, have antioxidant qualities that can aid in lowering oxidative stress in the liver. Vitamin D deficiency is common in people with liver cirrhosis, and it is crucial for bone health.

Dietary Guidelines for Liver Cirrhosis Patients

- **Protein Intake Recommendations**

High-quality protein sources include fish, poultry, eggs, beans, nuts, and dairy products. Emphasizing the consumption of certain meals is crucial. These sources provide essential amino acids needed for tissue repair and overall health.

Protein Restriction in Hepatic Encephalopathy: People with cirrhosis-related hepatic encephalopathy, which is characterized by cognitive impairment, may need to restrict their protein intake. This restriction is meant to lower the quantity of ammonia generated during the metabolism of proteins. A specific quantity of limitation is applied, taking into account the severity of encephalopathy.

- **Carbohydrates and Fiber**

Complex Carbohydrates: Give whole grains, fruits, vegetables, and legumes priority when it comes to complex carbs. These foods support general nutritional well-being and offer long-lasting energy.

Limit Simple Sugars: As they can aggravate illnesses like NAFLD and lead to weight gain, limit your consumption of simple sugars and refined carbohydrates. Keep an eye on blood sugar levels, particularly in diabetics.

Fiber Intake: Maintaining gut health requires consuming enough fiber. Whole grains, fruits, vegetables, legumes, and other foods high in fiber can help maintain regular bowel motions and stave against constipation.

- **Healthy Fats**

Focus on Unsaturated Fats: Give monounsaturated and polyunsaturated fats as well as other healthy fat sources top priority. Nuts, avocados, fatty fish (like mackerel and salmon), and olive oil are all great options. These fats can aid in the management of diseases like NAFLD and improve cardiovascular health in general.

Limit Saturated and Trans Fats: Cut back on the amount of processed foods, fried foods, and some cooking oils that contain saturated and trans fats. Reducing these fats can help maintain the health of the liver by reducing inflammation.

- **Micronutrients and Antioxidants**

Minerals and vitamins: Eat a varied and colorful diet to guarantee that you are getting enough of these nutrients. Antioxidants like vitamins C and E, which are abundant in fruits and vegetables, help prevent oxidative stress in the liver.

Sources of calcium and vitamin D should be included for the health of your bones. Bone density can be affected by liver cirrhosis, and these nutrients are necessary to keep strong, healthy bones.

Water: Those with cirrhosis, particularly those who experience consequences like ascites, must maintain adequate hydration. Reducing sodium consumption and maintaining proper hydration levels can aid in maintaining fluid balance and avert issues associated with fluid retention.

CHAPTER 5: MEAL PLANNING AND RECIPES

When it comes to managing liver health, proper meal planning is an essential component, particularly for people who are struggling with cirrhosis of the liver. When preparing meals that are suitable for the liver, it is important to give careful consideration to the nutritional content, portion sizes, and cooking methods available. This comprehensive guide will walk you through the process of preparing meals that are beneficial to the liver, provide a sample meal plan for seven days, investigate various cooking techniques that are beneficial to the liver, and offer a wide variety of recipes that cover breakfast, lunch, dinner, snacks, and desserts.

Building Liver-Friendly Meals

7 Days Sample Meal Plans

The health of the liver can be significantly improved by following a meal plan that has been carefully crafted. A sample meal plan for seven days is provided here, which emphasizes foods that are high in nutrients while also taking into account the particular requirements of those who have liver cirrhosis.

Day 1:

Breakfast:

- Tomatoes and spinach are added to scrambled eggs.
- Toast made with whole grains.
- Slices of fresh oranges.

Lunch:

- A chicken breast grilled.

- Salad made of quinoa and various vegetables.

- Greek yogurt with a honey drizzle.

Snack:

- Handful of almonds
- Apple slices

Dinner:

- Baked salmon with lemon and dill
- Steamed broccoli
- Brown rice

Dessert:

Berries mixed and topped with Greek yogurt

Day 2:

Breakfast:

- Strawberry slices and oats accompany a Greek yogurt parfait.
- A muffin made with whole grains.

Lunch:

- Soup made with lentils.
- Hummus on whole-grain pita bread.
- Salad of mixed greens dressed with olive oil.

Snack:

- Cucumber and carrot sticks served with tzatziki.
- Handful of walnuts.
- **Dinner:**
- Tofu stir-fried with snap peas and broccoli.
- Quinoa.

- mango slices.

Dessert:

- Chia seed pudding with sliced kiwi.

Day 3:

Breakfast:

- Kale, banana, Greek yogurt, and protein powder all combined into a smoothie.
- Bagel made with whole grains and cream cheese.

Lunch:

- Wrap made with whole-grain tortilla, turkey, and avocado.
- Berry salad mixed.

Snack:

- Pineapple chunks with cottage cheese.

- Handful of mixed nuts.

Dinner:

- Garlic and herb-infused grilled shrimp skewers.

- Greek salad with quinoa and roasted Brussels sprouts

- Dessert:

- Almonds dipped in dark chocolate

Day 4:

Breakfast:

- Mixed berries, almond milk, and overnight oats with chia seeds.

- Orange slices

Lunch:

- Brown rice bowl topped with salsa, corn, and black beans.

- Pair whole-grain tortilla chips with guacamole.

- Greek yogurt paired with honey.

Snack:

- Slices of fresh apple with almond butter.

- Dried fruit with trail mix.

Dinner:

- Fish baked with herbs and lemon.

- Asparagus and sautéed quinoa.

- With a balsamic vinaigrette, mix greens.

Dessert:

- Baked pear with cinnamon

Day 5:

Breakfast:

- Avocado mash and poached eggs on whole-grain bread.
- Segments of grapefruit.

Lunch:

- Chicken breast filled with spinach and feta.
- Quinoa salad topped with cucumbers and cherry tomatoes.
- Serve wholegrain crackers with hummus.

Snack:

- Fresh mango slices.
- Pistachios in a handful.

Dinner:

- Brown rice with vegetables stir-fried with tofu.
- Carrots and broccoli steam-cooked.

- Feta-topped Greek salad.

Dessert:

Yogurt with granola and mixed berries

Day 6:

Breakfast:

- Smoothie of bananas and blueberries with almond milk.
- A muffin made with whole grains.

Lunch:

- Quinoa bowl topped with roasted veggies, tahini dressing, and chickpeas.
- Cucumber slices served with tzatziki.

Snack:

- Kiwi slices with Greek yogurt.

- A handful of cashews.

Dinner:

- Quinoa salad with a Mediterranean flavor and grilled chicken kebabs.

- Sweet potatoes roasted.

- Mixed greens dressed with tahini and lemon.

Dessert:

- Pineapple sorbet

Day 7:

Breakfast:

- Omelets with cherry tomatoes and sautéed spinach.

- Avocado on wholegrain bread.

Lunch:

- Stir-fried vegetables and chickpeas over brown rice.
- Cucumber and tomato salad.
- Carrot sticks with hummus.

Snack:

- Slices of fresh pineapple.
- A handful of cashews.

Dinner:

- Tilapia baked with herbs and lemon.
- Quinoa and a medley of roasted vegetables.
- Lettuce mixed with a zesty vinaigrette.

Dessert:

- Yogurt parfait topped with mixed berries and granola.

Cooking Techniques for Liver Health

The best cooking methods can preserve the health of your liver while increasing the nutritious content of your meals. Think about the following techniques:

Baking and Grilling: Avoid frying and instead choose to bake or grill. Baking preserves food's natural characteristics without adding extra fats, while grilling adds a smoky flavor without using a lot of oil.

Steaming: A low-heat cooking technique that maintains the nutrient-dense nature of veggies and proteins. It's a great technique to cook fish, poultry, and veggies.

Cooking with Nutritious Oils: Use heart-healthy oils, such as olive oil, when sautéing. These oils offer necessary fats in moderation without endangering the health of the liver.

Herbs and Spices: Instead of using too much salt, add flavor to food by combining herbs and spices. Spices like ginger and turmeric, combined with herbs like parsley, cilantro, and mint, add flavor and may have anti-inflammatory properties.

Reducing Added Sugars: Choose natural fruit sweetness in dishes instead of adding extra sugar. This promotes liver health by controlling total sugar intake.

Portion Control: Take care of your portions to prevent overindulging, which puts stress on your liver. For those with liver cirrhosis, smaller, more frequent meals throughout the day could be simpler to digest.

Recipe Collection

Breakfast Options with Ingredients and Instructions

1. Avocado and Tomato Toast:

Ingredients:

- Bread made of whole grains.

- Mature avocado.

- Tomato slices.

- To taste, add salt and pepper.

- A poached egg on top is optional.

Instructions:

- The wholegrain bread should be toasted until golden brown.

- Spread a mashed, equally distributed ripe avocado over the toast.

- Place the cut tomatoes on top.

- To taste, add salt and pepper for seasoning.

- For an added protein boost, feel free to add a poached egg.

2. Berry Smoothie Bowl:

Ingredients:

- Mixed berries (strawberries, blueberries, raspberries)

- Chia seeds

- Granola for topping

- Greek yogurt

- Banana

Instructions:

Blend mixed berries, Greek yogurt, banana, and chia seeds until smooth.

Pour the smoothie into a bowl.

Top with granola for added crunch and nutrition.

3. Vegetable Omelette:

Ingredients:

- Feta cheese (optional)
- Fresh herbs (parsley, chives)
- Eggs
- Mixed vegetables (bell peppers, onions, spinach)

Instructions:

- In a bowl, whisk the eggs.
- Tenderize mixed vegetables with a sauté.
- Scatter beaten eggs over a pan of vegetables.

- Cook the eggs until they are set.

- Garnish with feta cheese and fresh herbs, if desired.

4. Overnight Oats with Mixed Berries:

Ingredients:

- Oats rolled.

- Milk with almonds.

- Various berries (blueberries, raspberries, strawberries).

- For sweetness, use maple syrup or honey.

Instructions:

- In a jar, mix almond milk with rolled oats.

- Add a variety of berries and use honey or maple syrup to sweeten.

- Store in the fridge all night.

- Savor your oatmeal cold in the morning.

5. Banana and Blueberry Smoothie:

Ingredients:

- Banana

- Almond milk

- Ice cubes

- Blueberries

- Greek yogurt

Instructions:

- Smoothly blend almond milk, Greek yogurt, banana, and blueberries.

- For a cool texture, add ice cubes.

- Serve right away.

5 Lunch and Dinner Recipes with Ingredients and Instructions

1. Grilled Chicken Quinoa Bowl:

Ingredients:

- Roasted vegetables (zucchini, bell peppers, cherry tomatoes).

- Grilled chicken breast.

- Quinoa.

- Lemon-tahini dressing.

Instructions:

- Cook the chicken breast completely on the grill.

- Follow the directions on the package to cook the quinoa.

- A range of veggies can be roasted.

- Combine quinoa, roasted veggies, and grilled chicken in a bowl.

- Pour in some lemon-tahini sauce.

2. Lentil and Vegetable Stir-Fry:

Ingredients:

- Cooked lentils.

- Various veggies (broccoli, carrots, snap peas).

- Lean protein of choice, or tofu.

- Ginger and soy sauce for taste.

Instructions:

- Tofu and a mixture of vegetables are pan-sauced.

- Include the cooked lentils.

- Add ginger and soy sauce for seasoning.

- Mix well until thoroughly blended.

3. Baked Salmon with Herbs:

Ingredients:

- Salmon fillets

- Olive oil

- Garlic clove

- Fresh dill, parsley, and chives

- Lemon slices

Instructions:

- Place the salmon fillets on a baking tray and preheat the oven.

- Sage salmon and drizzle with extra virgin olive oil.

- Top with slices of lemon.

- Bake the fish until it's done.

- Add minced garlic as a garnish.

4. Quinoa Bowl with Chickpeas and Tahini Dressing:

Ingredients:

- Cooked quinoa

- Cherry tomatoes

- Cucumber

- Tahini dressing

- Chickpeas

Instructions:

- In a bowl, mix the cooked quinoa, cucumber, cherry tomatoes, and chickpeas.

- Pour over some tahini dressing.

- Gently toss to combine.

5. Spinach and Feta-Stuffed Chicken Breast:

Ingredients:

- Feta cheese
- Garlic
- Chicken breast
- Fresh spinach
- Olive oil

Instructions:

- Turn the chicken breast into a butterfly.
- Add the garlic and sauté fresh spinach until it wilts.
- Stuff feta cheese and sautéed spinach into a chicken breast.
- Once the chicken is thoroughly done, seal it and bake it.
- Before serving, drizzle some olive oil over it.

5 Snacks and Desserts with Ingredients and Instructions

1. Greek Yogurt Parfait:

Ingredients:

- Mixed berries
- Granola
- Greek yogurt
- Honey drizzle

Instructions:

- Arrange granola, Greek yogurt, and mixed berries in a glass.
- Iterate through the levels.
- Before serving, pour some honey over it.

2. Nut and Seed Energy Balls:

Ingredients:

- Dates or figs

- Cocoa powder

- Almonds, walnuts, and chia seeds

- Coconut flakes

Instructions:

- In a food processor, blend nuts, seeds, and dates or figs.

- Add the coconut flakes and cocoa powder.

- Form into little balls and store in the fridge.

3. Baked Apple Slices with Cinnamon:

Ingredients:

- Cinnamon

- Nutmeg

- Apple slices

- Greek yogurt for dipping

Instructions:

- Apple slices should be arranged on a baking pan.

- Toss in nutmeg and cinnamon.

- Bake till just done.

- Accompany by serving with a Greek yogurt side for a dunk.

4. Hummus with Vegetable Sticks:

Ingredients:

- Carrot sticks

- Cucumber slices

- Hummus

- Bell pepper strips

Instructions:

- Place the veggie sticks on a platter.

- Accompany with a substantial amount of hummus for dunks.

5. Chia Seed Pudding with Mixed Berries:

Ingredients:

- Mixed berries
- Chia seeds

- Almond milk

- Maple syrup for sweetness

Instructions:

- In a jar, combine almond milk and chia seeds.
- When adding mixed berries, use maple syrup to sweeten.
- Chia seeds should be refrigerated until they swell and take on the consistency of pudding.

These recipes have been developed to provide a wide range of flavors and nutrients while staying conscious of the health of the liver. The preferences of the individual, any dietary restrictions, and any particular health concerns can all be taken into mind when making adjustments. Constantly seek the advice of medical professionals, including certified dietitians, to personalize meal plans and recipes to meet the specific requirements of each individual and to guarantee that they are in line with the overall management of liver cirrhosis.

CHAPTER 6: LIFESTYLE CHANGES FOR LIVER HEALTH

People who have liver cirrhosis should prioritize leading a healthy lifestyle to effectively manage their condition and ensure their overall well-being. One of the most important factors in maintaining healthy liver function is making certain adjustments to one's lifestyle, in addition to taking into account dietary factors and receiving medical treatment. In this all-encompassing book, we will delve into the significance of physical activity, provide advice for exercise, and investigate several strategies for stress management, such as yoga, meditation, mindfulness, and relaxation.

Importance of Physical Activity

Physical activity is an essential component of a healthy lifestyle, and the relevance of this component is magnified for people who have cirrhosis of the liver. Participating in regular physical activity confers a multitude of advantages, ranging from the enhancement of mental well-being to the improvement of cardiovascular health. Participating in physical activity that is healthy for the liver can contribute to several favorable outcomes, which are all related to liver health.

Exercise Guidelines

- Aerobic Exercise: Cardiovascular health can be improved by engaging in aerobic activities like cycling, swimming, or walking. Try to get in at least 150 minutes a week, spaced out across multiple days, of moderate-intensity aerobic exercise. This encourages improved blood flow and may help lower the chance of cirrhosis-related problems.

- Strength Training: Exercises focusing on strength are essential for those with liver cirrhosis. Concentrate on exercises with resistance bands or weightlifting that target your main muscle groups. Strength training helps to restore strength and muscular mass, which are frequently lacking in those with severe liver disease.

- Exercises for Flexibility: To preserve joint mobility and avoid muscular stiffness, incorporate stretches and yoga poses. Additionally, these exercises can help with balance, which is important, particularly if there is a chance of falling because of issues connected to cirrhosis.

- Consultation with Healthcare Professionals: It's important to get advice from doctors and physiotherapists before starting any kind of workout program. Depending on the severity of liver cirrhosis and certain medical conditions, they can offer tailored advice.

- Frequent Monitoring: Keep a close eye on how the body reacts to exercise and pay close attention to any indications of weakness, weariness, or discomfort. Exercise time and intensity should be modified according to each person's tolerance and health.

- Hydration: It's important to maintain enough fluids when exercising. Drinking enough water promotes good health and helps replace lost fluids through perspiration. This is especially important for those with cirrhosis who may need to manage their fluid balance.

- **Steer Clear of High-Impact Activities:** People with advanced liver cirrhosis should steer clear of activities that are high-impact and could cause harm. The health advantages of physical activity can be obtained without putting undue strain on joints through low-impact activities like swimming or stationary cycling.

Stress Management Techniques

- Stress and Liver Health: Prolonged stress can negatively impact liver function, making cirrhosis symptoms and complications worse. Promoting general well-being necessitates the use of stress management strategies.

- **Mindfulness and Relaxation**

The practice of mindfulness meditation entails developing an impartial awareness of the current moment. It can enhance general mental health and assist people in controlling stress and anxiety. Techniques like guided mindfulness sessions, body scan meditation, and deep breathing can be helpful.

Deep Breathing Exercises: Deep breathing techniques, such as abdominal or diaphragmatic breathing, help people relax and cope with stress. By using these techniques, you may fully expand and compress your diaphragm by inhaling slowly and deeply.

Progressive Muscle Relaxation (PMR) is a method of relaxation in which various muscle groups are systematically tensed and subsequently relaxed. This technique can reduce physical strain and encourage serenity.

Creating a mental image that encourages calm and good emotions is known as guided imagery. Imagining calm places or taking mental excursions can be effective methods for lowering stress.

- **Yoga and Meditation**

Yoga for Liver Health: Yoga is a holistic form of exercise that incorporates breathing exercises, meditation, and physical postures. Some yoga poses can be modified to help with flexibility, balance, and relaxation for those with liver cirrhosis. Pose variations that call for deliberate breathing and mild stretching might be especially helpful.

Meditation for Emotional Well-Being: Consistent meditation, whether it be transcendental meditation or mindfulness meditation, can improve emotional well-being. People who meditate regularly can develop a focused, serene state of mind that makes them more resilient to pressures.

Yoga Nidra for Deep Relaxation: Yoga Nidra, also known as yogic slumber, is a method of guided meditation that promotes profound relaxation. People with liver cirrhosis frequently struggle with sleep difficulties, therefore it can be very beneficial for them.

Including Stress Management in Everyday Activities: Try to be consistent in incorporating stress management practices into your everyday life. Regular practice improves the efficacy of these strategies, whether through quick mindfulness moments, deep breathing exercises, or meditation sessions.

Professional Advice: People who suffer from liver cirrhosis can think about consulting with yoga instructors or meditation specialists who are trained in helping people manage chronic illnesses. They can modify procedures according to the needs of each individual.

CHAPTER 7: MONITORING AND SUPPORT

Not only does providing care for those who have cirrhosis of the liver include proactive medical management, but it also involves providing essential assistance and monitoring on an ongoing basis. To monitor the progression of the condition and effectively manage any complications that may arise, it is essential to undergo routine medical examinations. In addition, supportive therapies, which may include involvement in support groups and the evaluation of mental health issues, are crucial components of a comprehensive approach to the treatment of liver cirrhosis.

Regular Medical Check-ups

- **Importance of Monitoring Liver Function**

The Need for Frequent Monitoring: Patients with liver cirrhosis must undergo routine medical examinations to evaluate their liver function, spot any problems, and modify their treatment regimens as necessary. By enabling quick intervention, monitoring helps healthcare providers avoid problems from getting worse and improves patient care overall.

Liver Function Tests: These vital indicators of the health and operation of the liver include measurements of bilirubin levels, clotting factors, and liver enzymes. Early detection of anomalies by these tests can help guide the therapy of cirrhosis.

Imaging Studies: Regular imaging tests, such as CT, MRI, or ultrasound, can be used to evaluate the liver's anatomy and spot any abnormalities, such as the existence of varices or ascites (fluid buildup) (enlarged blood vessels).

Endoscopy: The process known as esophagogastroduodenoscopy (EGD) involves looking within the stomach and esophagus. It is essential for diagnosing and treating varices, a potentially dangerous side effect of cirrhosis.

Assessment of Consequences: Routine examinations enable medical practitioners to assess cirrhosis-related complications, including ascites, kidney failure, and hepatic encephalopathy. Effective management of these problems is made possible by early recognition and prompt intervention.

Medication Adjustments: Monitoring offers a chance to evaluate the efficacy of drugs recommended for the treatment of liver cirrhosis. If adverse effects or changes in liver function occur, medication modifications may be required.

Vaccination Status: People who have liver cirrhosis must make sure they are up to date on their vaccines, especially those for hepatitis A and B. Regular examinations offer the chance to evaluate and update immunization records.

Monitoring Nutritional Status: For those with liver cirrhosis, monitoring includes determining their nutritional status. Healthcare practitioners can offer advice on dietary modifications depending on individual needs, as malnutrition is common in cirrhosis patients.

Patient Education: Routine check-ups provide an additional avenue for patient education. Healthcare providers can offer advice on changing one's lifestyle, managing symptoms, and sticking to treatment regimens.

Supportive Therapies

- ## **Support Groups**

The function of support groups is crucial in giving liver cirrhosis patients and their carers a sense of community, emotional support, and information exchange. By joining a support group, people can build a network of support and learn how to deal with the obstacles brought on by their illness.

Information Exchange: Support groups give people a place to talk about their experiences, perceptions, and coping mechanisms. People can feel less alone on their path and more empowered as a result of this information sharing.

Support on an Emotional Level: Managing a chronic illness can be emotionally taxing. Support groups provide a safe and understanding place for people to vent their emotions, worries, and frustrations. Making connections with people who are going through similar things can help you feel less alone.

Practical Advice: Support groups frequently offer helpful guidance on coping with cirrhosis on a day-to-day basis. This could include advice on managing symptoms, changing one's diet, and utilizing the healthcare system.

Support for Family and Caregivers: Support groups cater not only to liver cirrhosis patients but also to their relatives and caretakers. A support group can provide direction and understanding for caregivers as they navigate the enormous emotional and practical problems they confront.

Online and In-Person Options: People can choose to engage in support groups based on their preferences and location, as they are accessible through both online and in-person means. Accessibility is provided by online forums and virtual support groups, especially for people who might have trouble with mobility or transportation.

- ## **Mental Health Considerations**

Effects of Liver Cirrhosis on Mental Health: Mental health can be significantly impacted by having liver cirrhosis. Stress, anxiety, and sadness can be exacerbated by changes in lifestyle, the unpredictability of the illness, and possible complications.

Integrated Mental Health Care: In an integrated healthcare system, medical management and mental health issues are addressed together. To provide all-encompassing care, medical specialists—including hepatologists and mental health specialists—may work together.

Counseling and psychotherapy: To address emotional and psychological difficulties, people with liver cirrhosis may find it helpful to get counseling or psychotherapy. Coping mechanisms, emotional support, and a secure environment to discuss worries can all be obtained through therapeutic interventions.

Practices of Mindfulness and Relaxation: Including practices of mindfulness and relaxation in daily life can be good for mental health. Stress management and general well-being can be improved with methods like mindfulness meditation, guided visualization, and deep breathing.

Family and Social Support: Having a robust support system, comprising friends and family, is crucial for maintaining mental well-being. Maintaining open lines of communication with family members helps promote empathy and a supportive atmosphere.

Handling Isolation and Stigma: Feelings of isolation can be exacerbated by the stigma attached to liver disease. Any stigma-related issues should be addressed by mental health support, highlighting the fact that liver cirrhosis is a medical condition that calls for compassion and understanding.

Medication Considerations: People with liver cirrhosis may occasionally be administered drugs to treat mental health issues. Healthcare providers must take into account how drugs affect liver function and make the necessary modifications.

CONCLUSION

Recap of Key Points

The path to liver health is a complex one that calls for a mix of continued support, lifestyle modifications, and medication management. We have covered a wide range of topics related to liver cirrhosis in this extensive guide, such as its definition, causes, phases, and the critical role that nutrition plays in its management. A comprehensive approach to managing liver cirrhosis involves knowledge of the anatomy and function of the liver, common liver disorders, causes and risk factors, medical treatment techniques, nutritional strategies, meal planning, recipes, lifestyle modifications, and monitoring and support.

What Constitutes Liver Cirrhosis: Liver cirrhosis is a degenerative disease that leaves the liver tissue permanently scarred. It can result in decreased liver function and frequently arises as a consequence of chronic liver disorders.

The Stages of Liver Cirrhosis: Several stages of liver damage occur as the disease advances. Effective management of the illness depends on early discovery and action.

The Function of Food in Treatment: Nutrition is essential for managing liver cirrhosis. A diet rich in nutrients and well-balanced can help manage problems, improve general health, and support liver health.

Basics of Liver Health: Knowledge of the liver's structure and functions can help one better understand how the liver aids in digestion, detoxification, and the general management of liver diseases such as cirrhosis, fatty liver disease, and hepatitis.

Causes and Risk Factors: Several conditions, including non-alcoholic fatty liver disease, chronic viral hepatitis (B and C), and alcohol-related liver disease, can result in liver cirrhosis. Obesity and metabolic syndrome are examples of lifestyle factors that are also involved.

Medical therapy approaches include the use of immunosuppressants, antiviral medicines, and other pharmaceuticals. In more severe situations, surgical therapies such as shunt operations and liver transplantation may be explored.

Nutritional Techniques: These strategies emphasize the significance of following dietary guidelines, eating a balanced diet, and fulfilling nutrient requirements. Crucial components include controlling protein intake, selecting healthy fats, and making sure you're getting enough vitamins and antioxidants.

Meal Planning and Recipe Development: Creating meals that are liver-friendly requires giving considerable thought to the components and methods of preparation. For those with liver cirrhosis, a compilation of sample meal plans and recipes is available. These include breakfast options, lunch and dinner ideas, and snacks.

Lifestyle Adjustments: Including lifestyle adjustments, including consistent exercise and stress reduction methods, is crucial for general health. Holistic care includes instructions for exercise, awareness, relaxation, yoga, and meditation.

Monitoring and Support: It is essential to have routine checkups with a doctor to keep an eye on liver function, identify any issues, and modify treatment regimens. Supportive therapies offer emotional and social assistance. These include attending support groups and addressing mental health issues.

The Journey to Liver Health

Developing liver health is a dynamic process that calls for perseverance, dedication, and teamwork from patients, caregivers, and support systems. It is a customized journey that changes with time rather than a straight line. For the path to liver health, keep the following points in mind:

Tailored Care: The significance of personalized care is highlighted by the realization that every person's experience with liver cirrhosis is distinct. A more efficient and long-lasting strategy is guaranteed when medical therapy, dietary advice, and lifestyle modifications are customized to meet the needs of each individual.

Cooperation with Medical Professionals: The path to liver health begins and ends with a cooperative partnership with medical professionals. Effective management of liver cirrhosis can be facilitated by proactive and educated approaches, such as regular communication, openness about symptoms and concerns, and active participation in medical check-ups.

Empowerment by Knowledge: Knowledge is a potent instrument that enables people to actively participate in their health care. Comprehending the complexities of liver cirrhosis, its etiology, and the influence of lifestyle decisions facilitates well-informed decision-making and adherence to suggested interventions.

Adaptability and Resilience: These two qualities are necessary on the path to liver health. People may experience difficulties, failures, or unforeseen shifts in their health. A more proactive and positive journey can be achieved by adopting a resilient mindset and being flexible when treatment plans change.

Including Lifestyle Changes: Including lifestyle modifications such as a diet that is friendly to the liver, frequent exercise, and stress reduction methods is a process that takes time. Over time, small, sustained changes lead to long-term benefits for liver health.

Community & Support Networks: Creating a network of friends and family is an important part of the process. Support groups offer a sense of community, knowledge sharing, and emotional support. Developing a network of others who have gone through similar things as you do can help you deal with the difficulties of liver cirrhosis.

Taking Care of Mental Health: Achieving liver health requires taking mental health issues into account. A comprehensive approach to care includes treating mental health alongside medical specialists, obtaining help when necessary, and managing the emotional elements of living with a chronic condition.

Celebrating Progress: It's important to recognize and honor every advancement, no matter how tiny. There are turning points, advancements, and resilient moments along the path to liver health. Acknowledging and applauding these successes helps to maintain a positive perspective on the entire journey.

Sustained Monitoring and Adjustment: The path to liver health is a continuous one that calls for constant observation and modification. A proactive strategy for controlling liver cirrhosis includes routine check-ups with the doctor, modifications to treatment regimens, and keeping up with new advancements.

In summary, achieving liver health is a multifaceted and ever-changing process that takes into account lifestyle, food, and medical factors. People can overcome the difficulties and strive toward improving their liver health by being aware of the subtleties of liver cirrhosis, accepting tailored care, and developing a cooperative connection with medical experts. The path is made more complex by the addition of supporting therapies, community involvement, and an emphasis on mental health. This results in a holistic approach that takes into account the social, emotional, and physical elements of living with liver cirrhosis. Through empowerment, resilience, and sustained dedication, people can take a proactive approach towards liver health and improve their

general state of well-being.

www.ingramcontent.com/pod-product-compliance
Lightning Source LLC
Chambersburg PA
CBHW070853260726
48661CB00004B/1392